YOUR KNOWLEDGE HAS VALUE

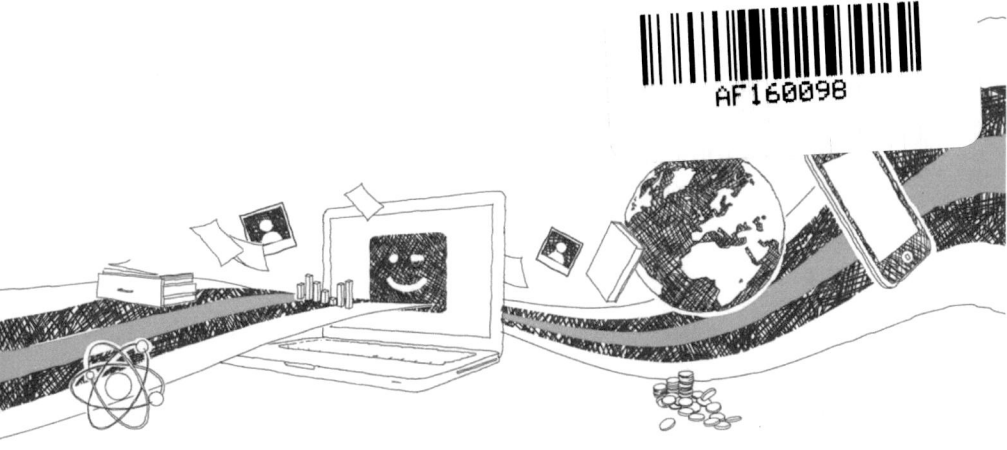

- We will publish your bachelor's and master's thesis, essays and papers

- Your own eBook and book - sold worldwide in all relevant shops

- Earn money with each sale

Upload your text at www.GRIN.com and publish for free

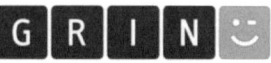

Bibliographic information published by the German National Library:

The German National Library lists this publication in the National Bibliography; detailed bibliographic data are available on the Internet at http://dnb.dnb.de .

This book is copyright material and must not be copied, reproduced, transferred, distributed, leased, licensed or publicly performed or used in any way except as specifically permitted in writing by the publishers, as allowed under the terms and conditions under which it was purchased or as strictly permitted by applicable copyright law. Any unauthorized distribution or use of this text may be a direct infringement of the author s and publisher s rights and those responsible may be liable in law accordingly.

Imprint:

Copyright © 2016 GRIN Verlag, Open Publishing GmbH
Print and binding: Books on Demand GmbH, Norderstedt Germany
ISBN: 9783668426672

This book at GRIN:

http://www.grin.com/en/e-book/356471/institutional-post-disaster-coordination-major-issues-and-insights-from

Bernice Debrah

Institutional post-disaster coordination. Major issues and insights from Nepal

GRIN Publishing

GRIN - Your knowledge has value

Since its foundation in 1998, GRIN has specialized in publishing academic texts by students, college teachers and other academics as e-book and printed book. The website www.grin.com is an ideal platform for presenting term papers, final papers, scientific essays, dissertations and specialist books.

Visit us on the internet:

http://www.grin.com/

http://www.facebook.com/grincom

http://www.twitter.com/grin_com

INSTITUTIONAL POST- DISASTER COORDINATION: AN INSIGHT FROM NEPAL

Bernice Debrah Graduate, Faculty of Health and Medical Sciences, Master of Disaster Management, University of Copenhagen, Denmark

Table of Contents

Abstract 3

Introduction 3

Methodology 4

Institutional coordination structures in Nepal 4

Coordination between national and international bodies 6

Major institutional coordination issues in Nepal (post-disaster situation) 8

Optimal level of institutional coordination: addressing issues in Nepal 9

Conclusion 11

Reference 12

Abstract

Coordination has been seen as a crucial factor in ensuring adequate response to disaster as well as successful reduction in future disaster risk. In light of this, the paper evaluated post-disaster coordination in Nepal. Secondary data was primary employed to review key relevant topics in post-disaster earthquake coordination. In the case of Nepal, a number of coordination challenges are evidenced in the strategic, operation and tactical level
A unified approach which incorporates all actors has been proposed for an optimal post-disaster coordination

Introduction

Nepal's location in the Himalayan- Alpine Belt makes it highly susceptible to various forms of man-made and natural hazards which often lead to disaster. In many of such large scale disasters, huge economic losses in the form of destruction of infrastructure and loss of lives are evident ("Disaster management reference handbook" 2015). It is commonly known that, the immediate consequences of disaster are judged by extremity of conditions. The situation's complexity results from the mere enormity of the urgency of the situation; Including factors like the provision of immediate relief and rescue support, challenges in accessing affected population, and the influx of interested stakeholders wishing to assist affected communities (ASEAN, 2008). All these factors need to be managed in a process that is timely and locally appropriate. Hence, coordination among both national and international bodies in post-disaster event becomes a crucial factor in ensuring adequate response to disaster as well as reducing future risk. In recent times, various collaborative efforts have been undertaken by international disaster management agencies to strengthen emergency operation and increase humanitarian response among countries and other agencies. All relevant stakeholders are required to have a shared goal, make a collaborative decision on actions to be taken and the procedure to attain those goals. Coordination plays a critical role in all these processes and refers to a deliberate action which seeks to harmonize 'individual responses' to ensure maximum impact (synergy) where the combined effect is greater than the sum of individual efforts (UNDAC Handbook, 2006). In the absence of effective coordination, inefficient use of resource, duplication of effort and dissatisfaction in response to affected communities is prevalent. Based on these, the paper seeks to propose an optimal level of institutional coordination for a post-disaster event in Nepal. Particular attention will be paid to coordination structures in Nepal, major post-disaster coordination issues and how such issues may be effectively dealt with at the strategic, tactical and operational levels.

Methodology

Secondary data was primarily employed to review major topics in a post-disaster situation. Key focus was on the coordination system in Nepal with key search relating to disaster coordination, coordination structures, earthquakes, emergency response, relief and cluster-coordination. Given that studies focusing mainly on Nepal's situation are limited in empirical studies, other sources including news blogs, relief organisation and government websites were employed.

Institutional coordination structures in Nepal

Various models of coordination structures have been institutionalized by the Nepal Government for managing disasters (Government of Nepal, ministry of home affairs, 2013; ("Disaster management reference handbook" 2015). The National Disaster Response Framework which is based on The Natural Calamity Act of 1982 guides the coordination as well as response activities between national and international bodies. In the context of this report, special focus will be placed on coordination relating to post-disaster events. The bottom up/down approach is used to coordinate activities at all government levels. On the strategic level, the Ministry of Home Affairs (MoHA) is the apex body mandated to manage immediate disaster response and recovery. It is required to serve as a linking agency between the National Disaster Management Agency (NDMA) which is yet to be established and the Nepal Government. Emergency Operation Centres (EOCs) have been set up at all levels of government administration by the MoHA with the National Emergency Operating Centre situated in Kathmandu Valley. In addition, various relief committees have been set up at all government levels. These committees are in charge of disaster response at each governmental level and are required to coordinate with each other. The Central Disaster Relief Committee (CDRC) which is headed by the Nepal Home Ministry is the next highest level in the coordination structure. Their major functions include coordinating activities of social organisations and mobilization of teams to assist in relief work in affected communities. The Regional Disaster Relief Committee (RDRC) performs similar functions as the CDRC but at the regional level. RDRC assists CDRC by reporting relevant information and implementing their directives. At the operational level, the District Disaster Relief Committee (DDRC) and Local Disaster Relief Committee (LDRC) perform relief and rescue work. In immediate response to emergency, DDRC deploys its search and rescue team with incident report to NEOC and MoHA as depicted in Figure 1. Once the CDRC recommends to the Cabinet for a declaration of state of emergency in response to a disaster event, specific activities are given to each of the various committee levels.

Figure 1: National institutional structures

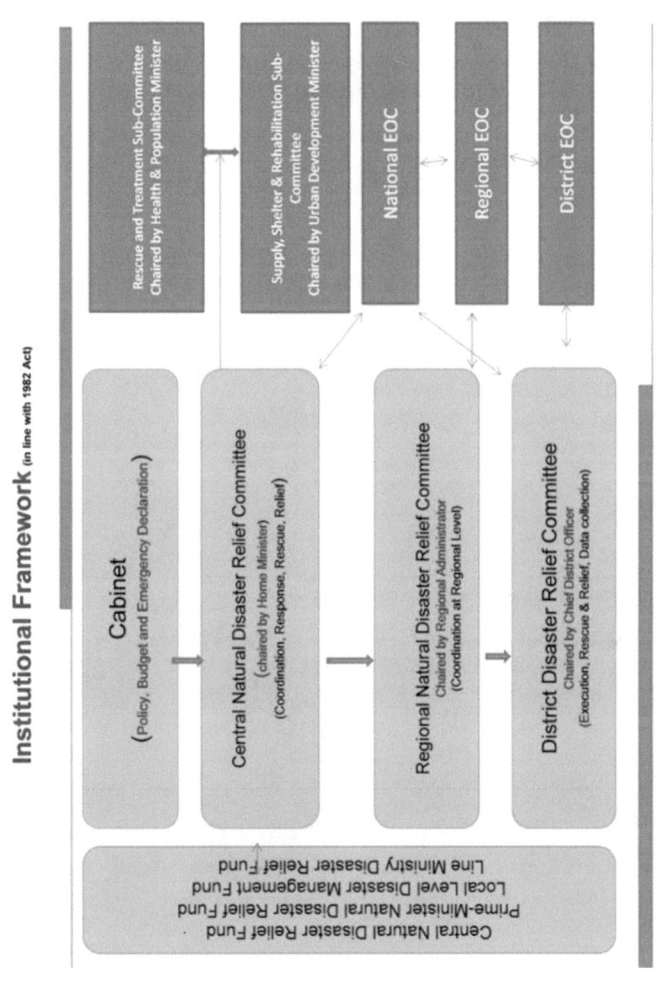

Source: Disaster reference handbook, Nepal (2015)

Coordination between national and international bodies

The cluster approach is incorporated into Nepalese coordination with international bodies (Government of Nepal, ministry of home affairs, 2013). Various ministries in Nepal are lead agency with the clusters as their Co-Lead (Figure 1). When capacity to coordinate in disaster is constrained or limited, a decision is made by the Nepal government to appeal for international support in kind or cash. The UN humanitarian Coordination of Nepal activates the various UN clusters once an appeal has been made. Coordination mechanism between the national emergency operation center and relevant bodies (military/On-Site Operation Coordination Centre (OSOCC), Multinational Military Operations Coordination Centre (MNMCC)) are automatically established in large scale disaster response (Figure 2).

Name of Cluster	Health	WASH	Shelter	Food Security	Logistics	CCCM	Education	Protection	Telecom	Nutrition	Early Recovery
GoN Lead	MoHP	MoUD	MoAD	MoHD	MoE	MoUD	MoE	MoWCS/ NHRC	MoIC/ WFP	MoHP	MoUD
Co-Lead	WHO	UNICEF	IFRC/ UNHABITAT	WFP/FAO	WFP	IOM	UNICEF/SC	UNHCR, UNICEF,	WFP	UNICEF	UNDP

Figure 2: cluster coordination structures in Nepal,

source: National Disaster Response Framework, Nepal (2013)

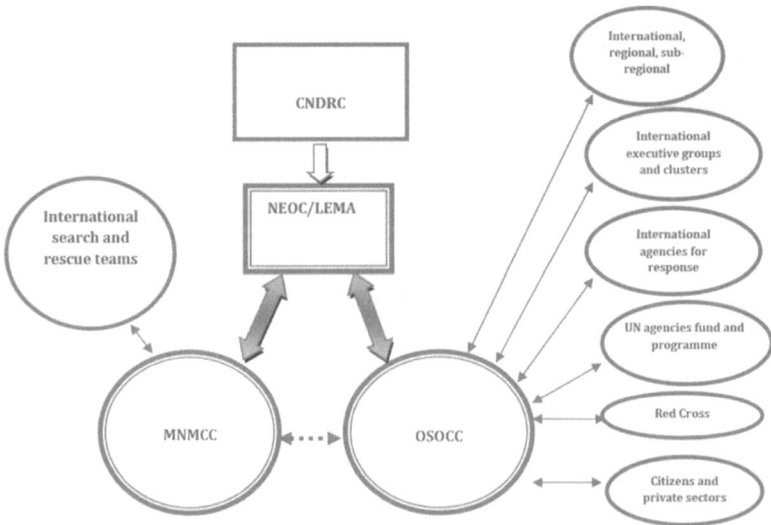

Figure 3: Coordination mechanisms between the national emergency operation centers
source:2 National Disaster Response Framework, Nepal (2013)

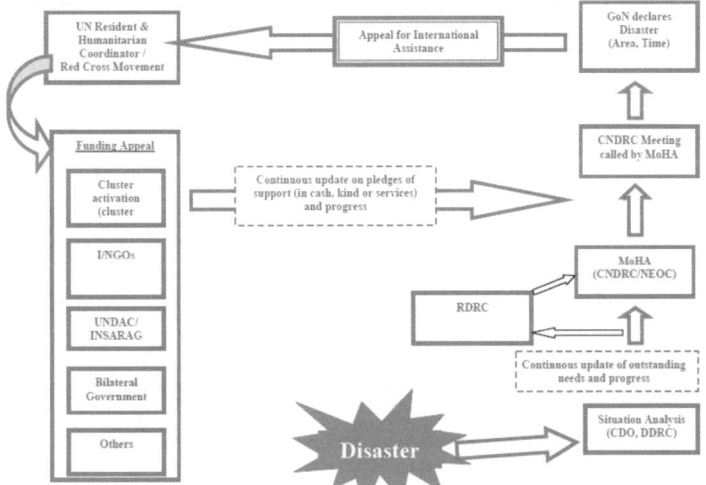

Figure 4: Disaster response framework
source: National Disaster Response Framework, Nepal (2013)

Major institutional coordination issues in Nepal (post-disaster situation)
Not much gap is seen in strategic coordination as there has been a huge investment in preparedness with training and simulation making it easy for the Nepal government to mobilize international, national and other voluntary bodies for the initial response phase (United Nations News Centre, 2015). However, in performing need assessment, a huge communication gap exists between higher government level (RDRC/ MoHA) and the affected communities at the grass root level (Village Development Committee (VDC) /Community Based Organisation (CBO)/beneficiaries). When disaster strikes, the local actors are usually the first respondent; National police and international bodies often arrive late(World Disaster Report ,2015). Situation analysis as depicted in the figure 3, often does not take into account concerns and needs of this group. This coordination gap could be attributed to the nonexistence of clear mechanism for communication (Nguyen, 2015). At the tactical level, the United Nations Office for Coordination of Humanitarian Affairs (OCHA) with the support of the Nepalese NEOC has played a key role with coordination of disaster response. However, inter-cluster coordination with national and local structures is often inadequate (Boersma et al, 2016). Activities of different clusters do not complement one another in achieving the overall agreed plan. Also internal coordination between civil societies agencies is also absent. The number of NGO/INGO has seen an increase in the past decades with the recent registered number standing at over 40,000 (Jones et al, 2014). Frequently the government's effort to coordinate international assistance has been overwhelmed as there is absence of a well-structured system to coordinate and monitor humanitarian assistance (Erica et al, 2015). The absence of effective coordination system between these bodies was evidenced in the recent earthquake where both the Nepalese government and the UN agencies made a separate appeal for funds. Even though reasons for such actions were attributed to the capability and credibility of government (Simon, 2015; trading economics, 2016), different agencies operating separately affected the overall cooperation and resulted in marginal rewards lesser than anticipated to beneficiaries. In addition, when international agencies and donors assume the role of the state, it affects the "Do no harm" principles. The "do no harm principles" is seen in many of such cases where external influences without direct government involvement has weakened the chain of accountability between the government and its citizens (OECD, 2009).On the ground of operations, transparency between government agencies (CB/VDC) and affected communities have reflected disillusion and disappointment with many feedback gaps. Often, beneficiaries not reached questions how funds are spent and why aid does not reach them. Various

programs have been established in attempt to bridge these gaps (Accountability lab 2016). The ability of communities to effectively communicate with government and the outside world will be important for effective rescue and relief effort. Furthermore, uneven distribution of NGO and duplication of relief activities have occurred, mainly attributable to an absence of mutual understanding and dialogue between civil society organizations (NGOs and INGOs) (Singh and Ingdal, 2007). Many smaller NGO failed to coordinate with each other; Often several agencies arrived at the same communities to addressed similar needs while other communities received no aid at all (Marson, 2015). Some NGO"s own interest and favouritism lead to absence of a systematic coordination. The UN humanitarian coordinator has been doing a great job on this part; however a coordination system where each agency's roles are well stated and incorporated into the overall goal can eliminate future gaps.

Optimal level of institutional coordination: addressing issues in Nepal

A unified approach which incorporates all relevant actors is necessary for ensuring optimal level of coordination. At the strategic level, a clear and concise communication system needs to be strengthened between existing government structures and grassroots level specifically among Community Based Organisations (CBO) and Village Development Committees (VDC) as these groups are not reflected in the national structures. As suggest by the world disaster report, local actors are usually the first point of call and therefore government agencies must incorporate their primary and secondary assessment input in the initial situational analysis. Every district is unique in its own way therefore local actors can better reflect the actual situation on the ground. Where Local actors and beneficiaries feel a part of the system, coordination is enhanced. Other initial assessments from NGO/INGO may also be included at this stage. To ensure effective tactical cooperation, there is a need for a strong inter-cluster coordination which factors existing civil societies (INGO/NGO) into collaborative mechanism. In achieving this, various INGO/NGO need to be designated to a specific co-lead cluster based on the goal of such organisation as depicted in figure 1. This will ensure effective placement of small organisation and resource optimization. Accountability to both Collective information systems need to be established among Cluster and Inter NGO which reflects beneficiaries needs. Duplication of effort can be totally eradicated in this manner with aid provided to the right beneficiaries. Traceability of funds would also be improved as it will ensure accountability to all parties involved. At the ground level, a clear medium for communication between beneficiaries, government and inter-cluster will be necessary to avoid loophole, rumour and contradictory messages. The bottom up approach will be essential in ensuring coordination at this level. Beneficiaries" feedback must be the ultimate goal at every stage to ensure accountability of financial aid. When trust is built, donors will have faith in the „Prime Disaster Relief Fund" as their aid will be guaranteed to reach the required beneficiaries. In the future, regional level structures need to be incorporated as semi-co-cluster leads to build more capacity within the national institutions. Regional levels relate directly with District and municipalities hence their input will help in fostering stronger force within the country. More importantly, local voluntary groups can be formed with team leaders recognized by Government bodies to keep the solidarity of Nepal citizens.

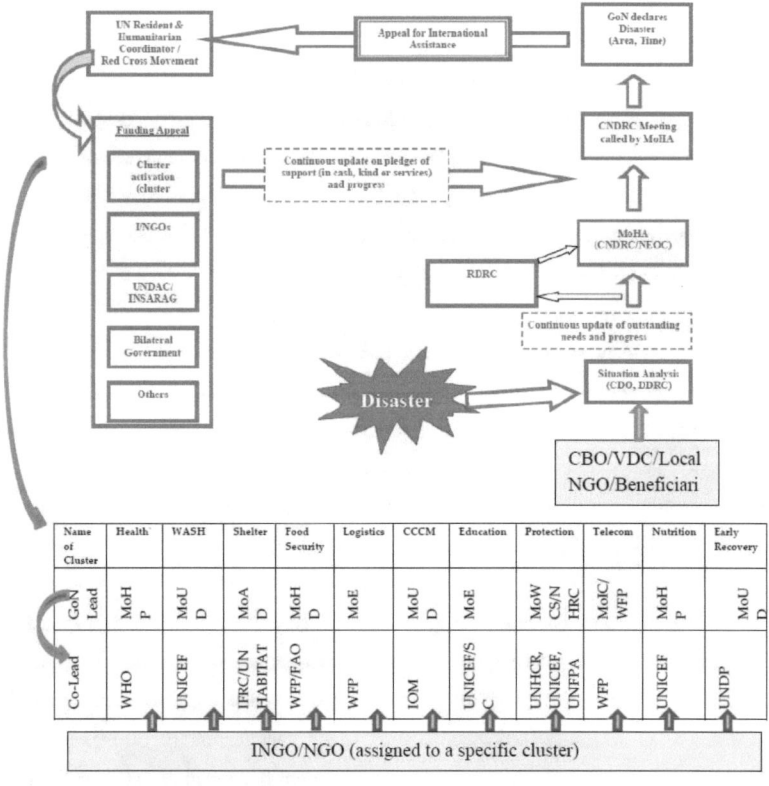

Figure 4: Proposed institutional post- disaster coordination structure

The figure was made by adopting existing response framework of Nepal and it cluster assignment structure. Researchers addition input has been made to propose optimal post disaster coordination. The green arrows represent coordination between respective bodies

Conclusion

The paper has addressed institutional post-disaster co-ordination issues in Nepal with focus on the 2015 earthquake event. Nepal institutional coordination structures were discussed as well as coordination between national and international bodies. Major coordination issues were evidence at the strategic, tactical and operational level. Given the challenges that arise in post-disaster situations, effective coordination mechanism must be enhanced at all levels with much focus on communities as they are the true beneficiaries. *"There is no emergency period where anything goes. Every response is either developmental or counter developmental; Every decision affects everything else."* (World Bank cited in Asian Development Bank, 2014). The decision taken is times of disaster contribute greatly to how affected community recover both in the short and long term. Therefore the suggestion provided above may be adopted to ensure a unified and cooperative approach in post-disaster events where future need are considered and previous gaps are avoided.

Reference

1. Accountability lab (2016). Nepal. Available at https://www.accountabilitylab.org/contry/nepal/ accessed on 27/09/16
2. Asian Development Bank. 2014. Operational Plan for Integrated Disaster Risk Management: 2014-2020.Manila. Available online at http://www.parkdatabase.org/files/documents/2008_Rapid-Damage-Assessment-and-Needs-Analysis-Manual_Quick-Reference-Guide_ASEAN.pdf. Accessed on 23/09/16
3. Boersma, F.K., J.E. Ferguson, F. Mulder and J.J. Wolbers (2016). *Humanitarian Response Coordination and Cooperation in Nepal. Coping with challenges and dilemmas*. VU Amsterdam: White Paper
4. Disaster management reference handbook Nepal (2015), Available from https://www.cfe-dmha.org/LinkClick.aspx?fileticket=xEUbtKHdfR4%3D&portalid=0 Accessed on 23/09/16
5. Erica, C.F., Lauren, B., Candice, S.A., 2015. Issues with Coordinating Aid Effort : Nepal Earthquake Clearinghouse. Nepal earthquake Clearinghouse. http://www.eqclearinghouse.org/2015-04-25-nepal/2015/05/06/issues-with-coordinating-aid-effort/ Accessed on 26/09/16
6. Government of Nepal, ministry of home affairs (2013) available from; http://www.ifrc.org/docs/IDRL/2011%20National%20Disaster%20Response%20Framework%20%28unofficial%20translation%20%29.pdf Accessed on 24/09/16
7. Jones S, Oven KJ, Manyena B, Aryal K. Governance struggles and policy processes in disaster risk reduction: A case study from Nepal. Geoforum. 2014 Nov;57:78–90.
8. Marson, A. (2015) Nepal Earthquake Recovery Appeal. Accessed on 4th November 2015. Available from:
9. http://bulldogtrust.org/wpcontent/uploads/2015/05/NepalEarthquakeRecoveryAppealStrategicOverview.pdf
10. Nguyen, Ly(2015). Communicating with communities a critical need in the humanitarian response to Nepal"s earthquakes IFRC Available from: http://www.ifrc.org/en/newsandmedia/newsstories/asiapacific/nepal/withcommunitiesacriticalneedinthehumanitarianresponsetonepalsearthquakes68849/ Accessed on 26/09/16

11. OECD, 2009. Conflict and Fragility Do No Harm International Support for State building: International Support for State building. OECD Publishing
12. Simoom cox (2015). Where is Nepal aid money going? BBC Radio 4"s The Report. Available from http://www.bbc.com/news/world-asia-3281774 accessed on 26/09/16
13. Singh, A., Ingdal, N., 2007. A discussion paper on donor best practices towards NGOs in Nepal .Norwegian agency for development cooperation (Norad), Oslo
14. The Association of Southeast Asian Nation (ASEAN)(2008), Rapid Damage Assessment and needs analysis Manual. pg. 4,. Available from http://www.parkdatabase.org/files/documents/2008_Rapid-Damage-Assessment-and-Needs-Analysis-Manual_Quick-Reference-Guide_ASEAN.pdf Accessed on 23/09/16
15. Trading economics (2016). , Nepal corruption index. Available from http://www.tradingeconomics.com/nepal/corruption-rank.Accessed on 26/09/16
16. UNDAC Handbook (2006), available from http://www.globalprotectioncluster.org/_assets/files/tools_and_guidance/natural_disasters/UNDAC_Handbook_2006_EN.pdf Accessed on 24/09/16
17. United Nations News Centre (2015). Nepal"s emergency preparedness saved lives in earthquake aftermath – UN health agency. Available from: http://www.un.org/apps/news/story.asp?NewsID=50844#.VjozyytSOpp. Accessed on 24/09/16
18. World Disaster Report (2015) Available from: https://ifrc-media.org/interactive/wp-content/uploads/2015/09/1293600-World-Disasters-Report-2015_en.pdf Accessed on 25/09/16

YOUR KNOWLEDGE HAS VALUE

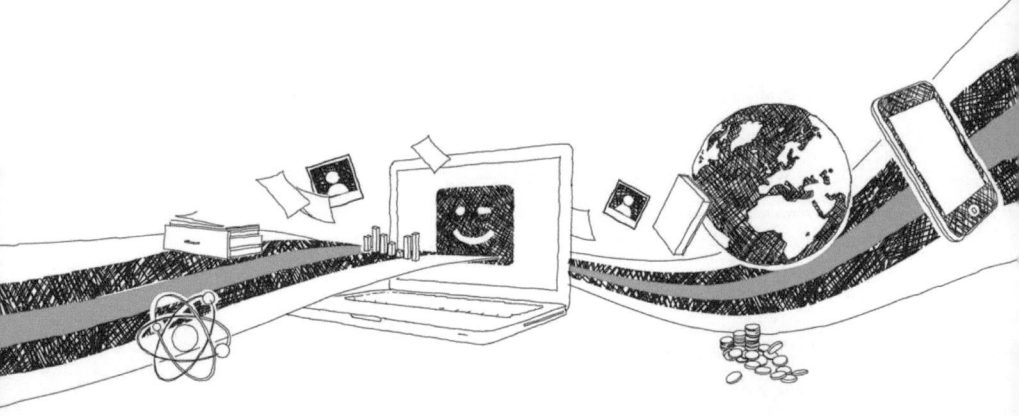

- We will publish your bachelor's and master's thesis, essays and papers

- Your own eBook and book - sold worldwide in all relevant shops

- Earn money with each sale

Upload your text at www.GRIN.com
and publish for free

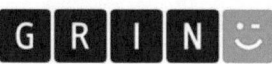